The Stay Young Revolution

How to Transform Fear of Aging Into Confidence of Youth

by

Martha Weinstein

with

Claire Fordham

ISBN-10: 1497327032
ISBN-13: 978-1-4973-2703-0

DEDICATION

For Rodrigo and Carlos and the many sons and daughters I recognize as such. You know who you are.

CONTENTS

MARTHA WEINSTEIN

FOREWORD

We've all heard the term "Renaissance Man" – someone with many talents or areas of expertise. Martha Weinstein is a Renaissance Woman. She seems to transform the ordinary into the extraordinary. She knows quality and class, but always elevates the uneducated and naive without her own ego needing the credit. Martha is a sage and ingénue at the same time. She tells it like it is, but with a positive point of view. She won't allow anyone under her wing to live from anything less than their strength. The generosity of her wisdom is her signature. Wherever she goes, she leaves beauty, strength, grace and intelligence.

Martha is also a shrewd businesswoman who can negotiate with the big boys. So the wisdom she shares is real-world, common-sense and inspiring. And she lives by the advice she gives. Martha has been a risk-taker, jet-setter, Latin entertainment icon and a trend-setter in the fields of beauty and anti-aging.

At a time when many Baby Boomers are facing illness, loss and loneliness, Martha teaches us to fish for an enhanced life in a clearer, fresher pond. This book is ice-cold water splashed in our faces. She wants us to wake up from long-held delusions by offering a different way of thinking: the secret of living congruently – attaining outward beauty and confidence from character and self-worth.

In this book, Martha extracts, condenses and communicates all the treasures learned from her own colorful and unique life, and the lessons gleaned from her clients and protégés. She knows women and how men relate to them. She knows human nature and how to balance work and play. If you take just one nugget from this book, it can change your life outside and inside.

We can all aspire to be like Martha Weinstein. She is sharing her method on how we can live from our own individual beauty every minute of every day, no matter our age. For that I am grateful. It truly is my blessing to have crossed paths with Martha and to have received her wisdom and elegance, along with the tools to feel confident and ageless with each passing birthday.

Dr. Aviva Boxer, OMD, PhD, LAC, HMD, CTN, ACN

ACKNOWLEDGMENTS

First of all, many thanks to Claire Fordham. More than just a ghostwriter, she is the force that moved the winds to this book being published. I also want to express my gratitude to my guardian angels and to the many friends and family members who encouraged me to keep writing.

Martha Weinstein

Working with Martha on this book has been an absolute joy. We first met when I was on the receiving end of one of her amazing non-invasive facelifts. As I listened to her stories of meeting Hitler, Mussolini and Peron when she was a child, I told her she really should write a book. She said funnily enough, she started one years ago and was looking for someone to help her finish it. I am so grateful to Martha for this opportunity, Colin Ryan for his editing skills, Joan Scheibel for the cover design and Diane Aldred for getting this book up, out there, typo-free and looking so fabulous.

Claire Fordham

www.clairefordham.com

www.joanscheibel.com

www.limetreestudio.com

MARTHA WEINSTEIN

INTRODUCTION

As I write this, I am eighty-nine years young and know I still have a brilliant future ahead of me. I am going to enjoy the rest of my life's journey.

The way I enjoy life is by helping others feel and look as young as naturally possible, at any moment in their lives. Forget about all those thoughts running through your head saying you're too old to live your dreams. You can do it. I am living proof.

An astrologer told me during a recent reading, "You are in this life to create a revolution. Not a political revolution, but a lifestyle revolution and you will write a book about it." She was adamant about it.

She talked about my previous lives and how those experiences play a part in who I am today. One of my hobbies is to make jewelry. In one of my oldest incarnations, I was the jewelry maker for the wives of a Chinese emperor. I was originally a man.

I have always felt I had the same potential as any man.

I thought, *That astrologer's right. I'm going to start a lifestyle revolution and share my conviction with as many people as possible that staying young is a lifetime's work, that you are never too old to start taking care of yourself and live your dreams.*

No one is ever too old or too young to join the "Stay Young Revolution." Let's change people's thinking and prove that there is always enough time to achieve what we desire.

Let's fight the prejudice, this belief system that takes the joy away from celebrating each birthday and embitters our potentially most fulfilling years.

If you want to mature youthfully, or if you ever thought that your life is passing you by without achieving your dreams, then this revolution is for you. Join me. Let's change the way people think and feel about getting older.

Long live the revolution!

1

THE RIGHT TO STAY YOUNG

A revolution is a form of liberation. When you have finished reading this book, hopefully, you will feel liberated from the chains of mental programming, negative patterns and limitations... all of them related to obsolete ways of thinking regarding what happens to a person with the passage of time.

I want you to be excited about finding ways to stay young, for yourself and for others. Research can be fun. Every bit of information you can use is a golden nugget you are panning.

Imagine yourself in the river, sifting sand and finding precious pieces of gold that will enrich your life forever. The same thing happens when you read a sentence that resonates in its wisdom and keeps shining in your mind like a beacon of light.

As revolutionaries, we are here to propose a new human right: The right to stay young. Yes, I'm proposing a right to stay young as part of the pursuit of happiness, which is meaningless without the exhilarating feeling of becoming wiser and more vibrant as time goes by.

Are you convinced you possess the right to stay young? To join this revolution, all you have to do is decide that you want to, and you're in. Are you in? Congratulations.

I want this to be a different kind of book. I want to start a conversation. Imagine you and I having a chat. It reminds me of when I had my television show in Argentina, coaching viewers to feel good about themselves. I was just talking into the camera, seeing only the lens, but knowing that they were on the other side in communication with me.

Do you want to find all the right ways to stay young? Of course you do.

You will know that you are winning the revolution when you get a feeling of fulfillment, enjoyment, creativity and peacefulness. You will learn that the most important thing is to always feel good about yourself. Not just for a little while, like the rush you get from eating chocolate or drinking coffee.

No matter what it takes or where it comes from, feel good about yourself.

So many people say, "growing old is such a bore." Too often I hear people say "I'm too old to do this" or "I'm too old to do that." Stop it now. Make a promise to yourself to stop negative thinking and speaking.

Tal Ben-Shahar teaches positive psychology at Harvard. He has proven that positive psychology is vitally important for humans. There's such a thing as an emotional IQ. Can you believe that?

Celebrating a new birthday should be enjoyable. I always celebrate each birthday for at least a week, if not more.

On my ninetieth birthday, I am going to dance the tango and there is a reason for it, as you will find out later.

All I ask from my fellow revolutionaries is for your cooperation. I jokingly say, "Be sensible, do as I tell you!" I have been doing this for more than sixty years and most of the time it works. It might sound a little too blunt, but I cannot be shy about saying things I'm sure will help. I promise you the process of change will be easier than you think.

My entire working life has been dedicated to bringing solutions to people about youthfulness, beauty and health. As I learned more, I realized I had to go deeper into the components of human happiness. Getting to know yourself and accepting yourself as you are is essential. Only then can you be helpful to others. And that's what makes life fulfilling.

A wise man said, "Love your neighbor as you love yourself." My answer to that is: start by loving yourself, then your neighbor.

When I propose that you join my revolution and be a Stay Young Revolutionary, an SYR, I am talking about real results, major improvements and true success stories. I have an obsession with results. This obsession is the fuel that drives my sense of fulfillment. It would make me extremely proud to obtain good results from making you a revolutionary.

In sport, a coach is necessary to help athletes achieve their potential. In everyday life, a coach or a mentor will support your desire to become the best you can possibly be and to feel good about yourself.

Today, a modern concept called a Life Coach has created

a new profession. Together with another modern concept called Wellness, it's possible to transform peoples' lives and worlds by changing the way they perceive their own realities.

I want to be your Stay Young Coach and explain all the basic things you need to slow down the ravages of time.

Remember my slogan, Be sensible, do as I tell you!

Let me describe what a Stay Young Revolutionary should be like. A revolutionary should have an attractive face, a healthy and shapely body, an open mind, good communicating skills and a compassionate heart.

But first, I need to tell you about my life so far and the experiences I've had that have made me the happy, healthy and youthful-looking woman I am today, and to tell you about the people I have met who have changed their looks in natural ways to make them feel and look better.

MARTHA WEINSTEIN

2

THE DAY I MET HITLER

I was born in 1924 in Argentina, the eldest child of an officer in the Argentinean army. My father, Bernardo Weinstein, was the only Jew in the Argentinean military to become a high-ranking officer.

My father was sent to Germany in 1935 to study strategy and tactics so he could go back and teach the subject as a professor at the Argentinean Military Academy.

The military world was divided between choosing to follow the British and American method or the German model. Argentinean military leaders opted for the German way.

My parents, sister, brother and I, along with our new German governess, boarded a steamboat for the twenty-day trip from Buenos Aires to Hamburg.

Once we arrived in Berlin, my father had diplomatic status, so we were protected by the law. This was extremely important in a country that was defying every possible notion of human rights.

My father wasn't a practicing Jew. He was open-minded about personal and religious choices, but the fact that we were in Hitler's domain was sensitive, to say the least. Most Germans had no clue what was going on and saw Hitler as a hero and a great leader.

Through the diplomatic courier, my father received Argentinean newspapers reflecting what was totally ignored by the German population: the disappearance of Jews from their homes and the existence of concentration camps.

Wealthy Jewish families were trying to escape by selling their valuables for very little and sending their money to faraway countries. Secretly, my father was helping in different ways. Because most of the actors of this drama are now dead, I feel it's OK to talk about it.

My father transferred money for Jews fleeing Germany to different countries so they had cash when they arrived at their destination. It was too dangerous for them to carry money with them, so he used his diplomatic channels to transfer funds in his name and put it in their names in their new bank accounts.

My mother also helped by buying furniture and silver from Jews fleeing Germany. She always paid market price. We had three containers the size of our living room full of items she bought to help people raise money for their safe passage out of Germany.

My mother was never happy in Germany. She didn't like socializing with the German wives or going to public ceremonies so, when my father was invited to the opening ceremony of the 1936 Berlin Olympic Games, he took me.

All the special guests and foreign diplomats were invited to see the beginning of the games from the main balcony with Hitler and his entourage, so I had the dubious honor of being introduced to Der Fuhrer.

I said, "Heil Hitler," the usual way of greeting, did my little curtsey then took my father's hand and we went back to our seats. I didn't look different to any other German twelve-year-old girl with little blonde tresses and a white summer dress.

I was there with all the German children saluting and

saying, "Heil Hitler." I had no idea what I was doing. People didn't say good morning or goodnight in Germany. Everything was Heil Hitler. So for me, saying Heil Hitler to Hitler was a normal thing as it was for all Germans. There was no consciousness attached to it.

A typical summer dress for young girls back then was a pale color with little flowers and a big splash of color across it. We wore our hair wound in tresses on either side of the face. For special occasions, the tresses were wound into two buns. That day, my tresses had a nice beige bow tied on at the end.

The happiest memory I have of the Berlin Olympics is that I saw the African-American Jessie Owens cross the finishing line and vividly recall him hitting the tape with his chest.

It was a delicate situation for the German government, because non-Aryans were considered inferior and not good enough to win. They had a hard time explaining how the black man was so superior.

Mr. Owens' victories didn't please Hitler, but Owens wasn't greeted with much fanfare when he returned to America either. President Franklin D. Roosevelt didn't meet and congratulate him as was the custom with returning Olympic champions. It wasn't until 1976 that his achievement was recognized when Gerald Ford presented him with the Presidential Medal of Freedom.

Anti-Semitism wasn't so noticeable to me and my family at the time of the Berlin Olympics. The Germans knew my father was Jewish, but our diplomatic status meant we were never affected by it. To the German officers, he was just an Argentinean major.

I didn't have a lot of contact with Germans. We mixed with other Argentinean officers and their families. I tried to be neutral. In the parks, there was a yellow bench for Jews, a green bench for the Germans who wanted to make a statement that they were against Jews and white marble benches for Germans who weren't anti-Jew. I chose to sit on the white marble ones.

My father's diplomatic immunity meant he could import anything he wanted. So he had an American car, a Hudson, shipped over. It was the only one of its kind in Berlin and people would stop in their tracks to stare at it. They assumed we were Americans. I identified with America, so when Jessie Owens won his four gold medals we were proud of him. An Argentinean woman won a silver medal in swimming. We were proud of her too.

I also met Benito Mussolini when I was a child. My family went to Italy and, as a visiting diplomat, my father had to present his credentials and pay his respects to the government. My mother, as usual, didn't want to go with him, so I went along.

An attaché introduced my father to Il Duce as "Major Weinstein of Argentina." My father bowed and said, "Viva Il Duce," the politically correct greeting of the time. I remember clearly that I wore a yellow summer dress. I kept my distance and stood by the attaché.

I thought Mussolini was ordinary, not at all charming. In fact, he was quite vulgar. Much different from all the other charming Italians I met. Maybe he was just playing tough to impress the Germans.

When I returned home to Argentina in 1938, I realized I had witnessed something special at the Berlin Olympics. Everyone was talking about how big an event it was. Germany was applauded for elevating the Olympics to such a prestigious international event. Hitler was still considered a good leader by most of the world.

Although Argentina didn't fight in World War II, my

family encountered obstacles when we went back and the leaders of the Argentinean military became pro-Nazi. With no explanation, my father was overlooked for promotion. There was a code of honor that you left the army if you weren't promoted. So my father had to resign his position in 1940, which broke his heart and began a difficult period in our lives.

My mother became very sick and had to have a kidney removed. Her illness was probably caused by the stress of my father's situation but, as always, some light was shone into our lives when my father was asked to participate in a new force called the Argentinean Gendarmerie, formed to protect our borders.

It was meant to be a security force of a military nature and my father's background was perfect to help establish this new organization.

My father brought home swatches of fabric for the new uniforms and because he was color-blind he asked me to select the shades for the jackets and trousers. To this day, the officers and sub-officers of the Argentinean Gendarmerie are wearing the colors I chose when I was fifteen years old, more than seventy years ago.

I never personally had a problem being Jewish in Argentina. There were anti-Semitic outbursts and some people I know suffered, but, apart from my father being overlooked for promotion, we never did. I had an identity card that described me as the daughter of a military officer and it opened all doors for me as if by magic.

When I found out about the Holocaust, I was deeply shocked and to this day I cannot bear to think about it. I haven't visited the Museum of Tolerance here in Los Angeles where I live now, because it breaks my heart.

I have witnessed many interesting events in my life and met some of the most powerful people in the world. I first met Evita (Eva Peron) when she was still an actress and not the influential person she became. The Argentinean people started calling her Evita when she became a leading advocate for the poor. I think it was part of a marketing exercise. It made her sound more saintly.

My Physical Education class visited the film studios where she was shooting a movie. When Evita married the then Colonel Juan Peron, who became Argentina's feared dictator, she had all her films and her birth certificate destroyed. She didn't want to be remembered as an actress, only as the savior of the poor.

Evita wasn't particularly good or famous as an actress. She was an escort who became an actress under the patronage of some other military men she befriended. Like the geishas in Japan, sex wasn't necessarily part of the arrangement.

As students, we were forced to attend public occasions and cheer for the Perons. I felt sorry for her. She was deeply resentful that she came from the wrong side of the tracks.

Evita's mother was never married to her father. In Latin America, it was common for men to have "the little house" where their lovers and their children lived. They kept their main family for official appearances completely separate.

Evita's mother was the mistress of a powerful industrialist and landowner. When he died, his mistress and their five children, including Evita, couldn't attend his funeral because they were bastards – a great stigma in those days. Evita hated everything to do with the establishment and wealthy people in general. I believe she helped the poor as a pretext for disowning the rich.

I don't think Evita was madly in love with Peron, but I think she was impressed by him. He was charming and could turn it on whenever he wanted. He was always nice to me when I met him. But when he became a dictator, he wasn't so delightful. He had been a school friend of my father and they sat next to each other in class. They even went to military school together. They were personal friends, but political adversaries.

My father belonged to a well-established political party, the "Radicales" — like the Democratic Party in America — and when Peron created his own party, he asked my father to join him. But my mother wouldn't allow it. She said, "Me? Sit next to that woman? Never!"

As for Peron, after my father explained his political reasons for not joining his party (not mentioning my mother's remarks, of course), he acted like a true friend and reinstated my father in the army with the rank of Lieutenant Colonel and a higher pension, then appointed him a counselor in the defense of the borders. We all recovered our peace of mind and I pursued my career as a mentor for women.

3

LOVE AND PASSION

My mother, Elvira, adored my father, but she wasn't warm and affectionate to her three children. We were just a by-product of her relationship with him. She also felt that having children was her duty to society.

Mine was not a happy childhood. It was challenging in many ways. I didn't have easy access to my mother and always had to deal with nannies and governesses.

My earliest memory is aged two months, when my mother came to the ladies' room at a social club to breastfeed me. My nanny handed me to her and she fed me as quickly as possible so she could get back to dancing the tango with my father. If you were wondering how I managed to recall such detail, I did regression therapy during psychotherapy as an adult and relived the moment. I believe my asthma was triggered because my mother was always in such a hurry to feed me.

Later, I tried a re-parenting technique where you can relive the feeling of being loved, cuddled and wanted by your parents, even if that didn't actually happen when you were a child. I found it powerful and effective.

My mother was a great beauty. A little heavy by today's standards, but she had a pretty profile and beautiful blue eyes. I inherited that tendency toward heaviness and my mother's unshapely legs!

She used Elizabeth Arden make-up and beauty products for many years, having been brainwashed into believing they were the best after visiting the Elizabeth Arden Institute in Paris. It was a huge validation for me when my mother started using my products instead. Finally, I was getting support from her too.

My mother was also a pioneer. At eighteen, she was one of a few women who entered university to study philosophy and literature. She graduated with a degree, specializing in ancient Spanish literature.

Susana, our brother Hugo, and I were familiar with the Classics from a young age. Elvira made us read them aloud so we could practice the power and joy of reading poetry in public.

There was no television in those days, and movies were just starting, so people had to entertain themselves. At parties, someone would play the piano, another sang, another danced and my mother recited poetry. That's what she loved doing the most.

Unusually for the times, my mother continued to work, as a professor of literature, after she married my father at twenty-three. She was also a school principal for a brief period.

My parents were very much in love. They were so happy together. The only thing that mattered to my mother was to keep my father happy, and to keep him away from trouble and temptation. She thought she was the salt of the earth and convinced my father she was too. My father, who was four years older than her, was in heaven.

They spent their fiftieth wedding anniversary dancing the tango because that's what they were doing when they met. I was born ten months after my parents married. They danced together every weekend until my father died, aged eighty-six. Mother died six years after him, aged eighty-eight.

Everything had to be done my mother's way. I'm a Scorpio and I like things to be done my way. So I was often in conflict with her. But I adored my father. I felt I had failed him by being born a girl. A son would carry on the family name, so I decided to keep my maiden name and make the family name as well known as a son could do.

It gave me a big thrill when my father was referred to in a newspaper article in Argentina as "Lieutenant Colonel Weinstein, father of the famous Martha Weinstein" and I was making a lot more money than him. I thought to myself, *mission accomplished*.

With such a strong woman for a wife and an unusual (for the times) respect for women in general, it's no surprise my father always supported me in whatever I wanted to do. In the 1950s and '60s in Argentina, women were still second-class citizens. It became my goal to support women's causes and encourage Argentinean women to be more independent, especially financially.

So I followed two careers. I went to law school and I studied physical education at degree level.

One career was to nurture my intellect and prepare me to

be a defender of women and children, the other to create a strong and healthy body and have a career educating others to do the same.

In those days, very few women attempted to enter law school and the examiners were especially hard on them. It took me three attempts to pass the test and I only prevailed the third time because I made my father come to witness the exam. They did not dare to intimidate me with my military father in the room. Everyone knew him. My answers were correct and I passed.

Physical Education had an easier exam and many girls were applying to a school that had separate programs for men and women. The good thing about law school was that I could pick and choose my dates among the male students as I was one of the few women attending.

The bad thing was that the way law was practiced in my country made it profoundly unappealing to me. As an attorney, I wanted to be the knight in shining armor defending the underdogs: women and children.

But it was all about pushing papers in moldy little rooms. There were no courtrooms full of life and characters like in the movies, or dramatic oral arguments. Just battles fought over typing machines and lots of filing.

Yet physical education was absorbing, demanding and lots of fun, so I abandoned law school, kept some of the friends I made and decided to help women and children by making them beautiful, healthy and strong.

At twenty-one, I opened my own little gym in the best part of town working with a private clientele receptive to my style of training. I was the first local trainer to create an exercise program for pregnancy and post partum that became a trend in itself.

It was a big joke in my family that at twenty-two I was making more money than my father. But life had other plans for me. It was the early days of television and I was offered the chance to teach exercises on TV. I had the two most beautiful models in Argentina as my demonstrators.

I wrote a best-selling book, *Remodeling Gymnastics*, and became a household name. Not many people had TVs in those days, but those who did only had one station. If people wanted to watch television, they had to watch me.

I received so much publicity that Martha Weinstein became a well-known brand – this was in the days long before branding was a buzzword. The network allowed me to do whatever I wanted on my show and I started to include everything related to beauty and self-esteem.

The show didn't run during the summer, so while it was off the air I traveled all over the world, taking courses on personal growth and aesthetics. I went to France, Italy, Switzerland and the United States, and took everything I learned back home. I became the Argentine Oprah.

My program was part talk show and part reality. A popular segment was Miss Cinderella that was all about transformation. During the first series, Miss Argentina was selected as a direct result of the Miss Cinderella segment. People sent in their photographs and we held a lottery to select the winner who we filmed going through the transformation process – everything from hair and make-up to teaching them about exercise and lifestyle. I even introduced plastic surgery.

I understand plastic surgery helps people who have no other choice if they need to correct a deformity, but I wouldn't recommend taking such a big risk exclusively for reasons of vanity.

There are so many negative aspects. It can be really painful and take a long time to heal. You are never the same person and often people don't look how they had hoped after it. And, of course, when faces are pulled and lifted, people no longer look like themselves and it can affect them psychologically.

I learned to distrust plastic surgery after all the bad examples I saw. As my confidence grew, I had the courage of my convictions to speak out against it. I prefer a natural look. I have never had plastic surgery and I never will.

Even so, it was a big advertising opportunity for the dermatologists and plastic surgeons who came on my show, as well as the hairdressers and make-up artists, and everyone else in fashion. The closing segment was a small fashion show, called The Runway.

We were on the air twice a week and, little by little, the program expanded into a talk show about beauty and self-esteem that lasted close to twenty years on Channel 7.

A few years ago, I went to the consulate to renew my Argentinean passport. The clerk said, "Wait a minute while I see if the consul is here so he can sign your passport and you won't have to come back to pick it up."

I waited patiently and the consul himself came out. He said, "Martha Weinstein? You have no idea how important you have been in my life. From the time I was eight years old, my mother wouldn't let me budge while your program was on the television. I lost my mother when I was fifteen, so all my time spent with her was precious and anything that made her happy made me happy. From now on, you will be treated as a VIP here. I just love you."

Things like that happen to me all the time. After many years on the air, you do reach a lot of people. Some of those people now live in other countries and I meet fans of my show all over the world. Many of my former students are reconnecting with me on Facebook. You have to keep up with the times in the Stay Young Revolution.

When I started living a public life, my maternal grandmother, Rebecca, didn't approve that I kept my maiden name after I married. She thought it was too bold for a decent woman. Rebecca was controlling, quite an icon herself. She was president of many Jewish charities in Argentina. She considered me the black sheep of the family.

Years later, she said to me, "Of all my grandchildren, I am proudest of you." So my greatest hopes were fulfilled: the approval of my father, mother and grandmother. Grandma Rebecca's approval was my greatest achievement. She was the mother of all generals.

I attended a party in Buenos Aires for visitors from Europe (who were in the country buying trees to grow for paper). So many languages were being spoken. At that time, I was seeing a tall, dark and handsome Italian who took me to the party.

A friend had advised me to be careful. Because this man was the type of guy who takes you to a party, abandons you and womanizes all night, then, at the end of the party, comes back to you and says, "Let's go home."

I said, "OK. I've been warned."

We arrived at the party, he introduced me to the organizers and off he went. I looked around and saw another handsome guy. It was a fancy dress party and we had to dress up in something that represented Argentina. You were either a Gaucho or an Indian, or something like that.

This guy was wearing the boots, pants and a beautiful silk shirt of a landowner. The shirt was monogrammed with his initials, A.I. He approached me with a drink in his hand and said in English, "What language shall we speak?"

"Any one you like," I said.

I spoke six languages and thought that was enough. It wasn't. He spoke many more.

"Then let's speak Warunee." It's the language of a small tribe of Indians in remote northern Argentina. He knew how to speak it because he had lived there.

"I'm sorry," I said. "You've got me. I don't speak Warunee."

"So let's dance the tango."

Another passion of mine is the tango. No other dance is more passionate. As the great Argentinean writer Jorge Luis Borges said, "It's a sad song you can dance to." When a couple dances the tango, they are embarking on a romance. The man is definitely the one who says how the dance is going. The woman is more submissive and it becomes an intimate relationship.

I danced with him so passionately I broke the heel on my shoe. I danced the rest of the night stepping on his feet, but we kept going and he was the life of the party. He played the accordion. He played the piano. He sang. He entertained the partygoers all night.

At the end of the evening, he said, "Would you allow me

to take you home?"

"I came here with somebody," I said.

"I don't see that somebody taking good care of you."

"You're right. You can take me home." After dancing the tango with this guy I would have followed him anywhere.

Alberto Iglesias was thirty-six and I was thirty-two. He took me to his home and we became a devoted couple.

He made a good living as a cosmetic chemist, but he was also an adventurer, as well as a wonderful writer who had won many literary awards in Argentina. I was independent, had my own business and traveled a lot. We clicked.

We belonged to a club called the Happy Divorcees. I had been married briefly before and Alberto had been married twice. We had many wealthy friends, one of whom had a penthouse in Buenos Aires and was always organizing parties for divorced people. One day we were in the elevator going up to the penthouse for a party and I turned to Alberto and said, "What must people think about us? We're always coming to these parties together, but we're not explaining why."

"We could tell them we are going to get married."

"But that's a lie."

"Maybe it's not."

"Is this a proposal?"

"Yes."

"What about children?"

"No children."

"OK," I said. "When would this marriage be? Maybe in six months?"

"I think two months is long enough to wait."

We were married two months later.

My husband was such an interesting person, highly intelligent and well read. We would talk about T.S. Eliot, all the great poets and the right way to read them aloud.

We talked about politics. Alberto was part of the failed revolution to overthrow Peron. Some of the revolutionaries were caught and disappeared. He was lucky. We talked about history, travel, literature.

He would tell me about his incredible adventures. Alberto was considered the Argentinean Hemingway. He lived in the rainforest for several years, writing his books and hunting and fishing to feed himself and his eleven dogs.

Alberto would stay at home writing and when I came in from my work, the most important thing was for me to read aloud what he had written during the day. He didn't believe in what he was writing until then. My mother's training to read the Spanish classics in public was excellent preparation.

This created a deeply intimate relationship between us. As a cosmetic chemist, he also went to our manufacturing plant and created the products I was selling on TV. He would bring home hundreds of different samples and give each one a funny name just for us to use. One was called Pig Pink, because it was the color of a little piglet. All the products had a fun name as well as an official name.

We had all this fantastic creative time with the products, his books and expanding the business. We had so much in common.

Then Alberto's son from his second marriage showed up one day at our business looking for his father. Carlos was a handsome, beautiful, adorable boy of sixteen but Alberto wasn't keen on children of any age.

I said to Alberto, "You're going to kick him out? You're crazy. I'm taking care of this child."

So I helped Carlos Iglesias start a career as the best-paid, most famous male model in South America. He was the Latin American Marlboro Man. He was so very handsome and professional, always punctual and immaculate.

I considered Carlos my son, but I was thirty-six and my biological clock was ticking. Alberto still didn't want to have children, but now I did. I told him about my change of heart and he said, "Well, our agreement was no children."

"OK, then we'll separate because I want a child. I have to look for my child's father."

He couldn't believe it, but I did it. I went back to my parents' house and started looking for the father of my child. And I found a man who wanted to marry me and have a child with me.

He was the principal where Carlos went to school. He was amazed how good a mother I was to my stepson and how well I managed his life. He said, "I will have a child with you."

Two months later, Alberto came crawling back. He had lost twenty pounds and was miserable. He said, "I can't live without you. I'll do whatever you want."

I explained to the principal that I was returning to my husband because I had a long history with him and he was dying without me. He took it very well and we parted on good terms.

I said to Alberto, "First you have to find us a nice place to live," I said. "And then I want to get pregnant."

Alberto didn't care about the school principal so long as he had me back. He found a beautiful condo in a nice area of the city and I went back to him.

We went to an auction and I bought a picture of a boy wearing a little pointed hat, playing the flute. I said, "I'm going to hang it in our living room. It will be the inspiration for our child. I want a Leo baby because Leos are good children to their parents. Then maybe if I'm not a good mother, he will be a good child."

I timed things perfectly and our beautiful son Rodrigo was born a Leo. I walked into the delivery room, had a natural childbirth and walked out pushing my baby in a cart. I was the happiest woman in the world.

And a pioneer as well. In those days in Argentina, women usually took painkillers and anesthetics during childbirth.

Against all odds, Alberto was the best father, because this child didn't cry and slept soundly at night so Alberto could concentrate on his writing. Rodrigo was so sweet that Alberto fell in love with him. He adored Rodrigo. Our life was blissful until Rodrigo became sick with kidney problems and we devoted our lives to making him well.

For six years, between ages two and eight, we let others run the business and just cared for him. The doctors told us we would never know if he would live to eighteen, the age when his kidneys would be fully developed.

The doctor also said, "If you have another child, this one will die because there is no way you can take care of him the way he needs to be taken care of."

So we didn't have another baby. But we had Carlos, so we had two sons and Rodrigo became strong and healthy.

When he was sixteen, Rodrigo was expelled from high

school for being rebellious, three months before graduation. So I went to the old school Carlos had attended and said to the principal (the man who had offered to marry me and father my child), "I need you to help me with my son and allow him to come to your school so he can graduate."

The principal had never married. I think he was still in love with me and wanted to help me as a friend. He didn't say he was still in love with me, but a woman can tell these things.

Rodrigo wasn't a bad child, but he said his old school principal was a tyrant who was way too strict, so he refused to obey all her many rules and regulations. I went to talk to her, but she said there was nothing she could do.

Sitting at our family dinner table, I was providing the stage and directing the transit between three vastly different personalities who were always meeting for lunches on weekends and dinners on weekdays, where there was a lot of love and competition at play. Number One: the writer, poet, chemist. Number Two: the elder son, model and TV personality. Number Three: the young Leo, the protected one. Dealing with issues of all kinds kept my mind exercised and flexible.

Alberto and I were together for twenty-five wonderful years until he died of a heart attack.

Carlos is now seventy and Rodrigo just turned fifty. The brothers are extremely close and love each other very much. They are both wonderful sons. Carlos lives in Argentina, but emails me twice a day and visits me often. Rodrigo lives in Malibu.

I was always Martha Weinstein, never Martha Iglesias. My husband had no choice. He married a woman with a purpose. He loved the fact that I was independent and had my own approach. Without being a feminist, I was pro women's rights and pro women's choices.

Another great love for me was my sister, Susana. We lived together in the United States for several years. To come home to someone you love is a wonderful thing. Susana and I ate dinner together every night, went to the movies and traveled the world. We adored each other. My time living with Susana was one of the best of my life.

Susana was misdiagnosed in America with Parkinson's Disease, but I took her back to Buenos Aires and she was put on the right medication to treat her dementia. When she got sick, it was a painful time to watch her decline.

Susana lived in a good clinic in Buenos Aires and her adoring daughter, my niece Gabriela, took daily care of her. I visited twice a year until she died aged eighty-one, two months after my eighty-fifth birthday. I celebrated that birthday in Argentina. I made it a lunch party so she could be there. She arrived in a wheelchair and seemed to recognize everyone. I have beautiful memories and treasured photographs of that birthday.

Now I live alone and miss Susana so much. It brings me great comfort that she didn't suffer at the end and died peacefully in her sleep. That's what I wish for myself every time I blow out a candle on my birthday cake. I make a wish to die like my sister. But not for a while.

Our baby brother Hugo is eighty-one (at the time of writing this) and lives in Orange County, California with his magnificent wife, Norah, and lots of children and grandchildren. When I see Hugo and Norah, we have fun together and catch up on gossip. I am lucky to have a big, wonderful family.

Not everyone is blessed with good genes, children, or the joy of a great and passionate love, but it is vital to have love and passion in your life, whether it's the love of a faithful companion, good friend, hobby, charitable work, or a great and rewarding career.

Now my passion is my work. Please, find something or someone to love and be passionate about.

MARTHA WEINSTEIN

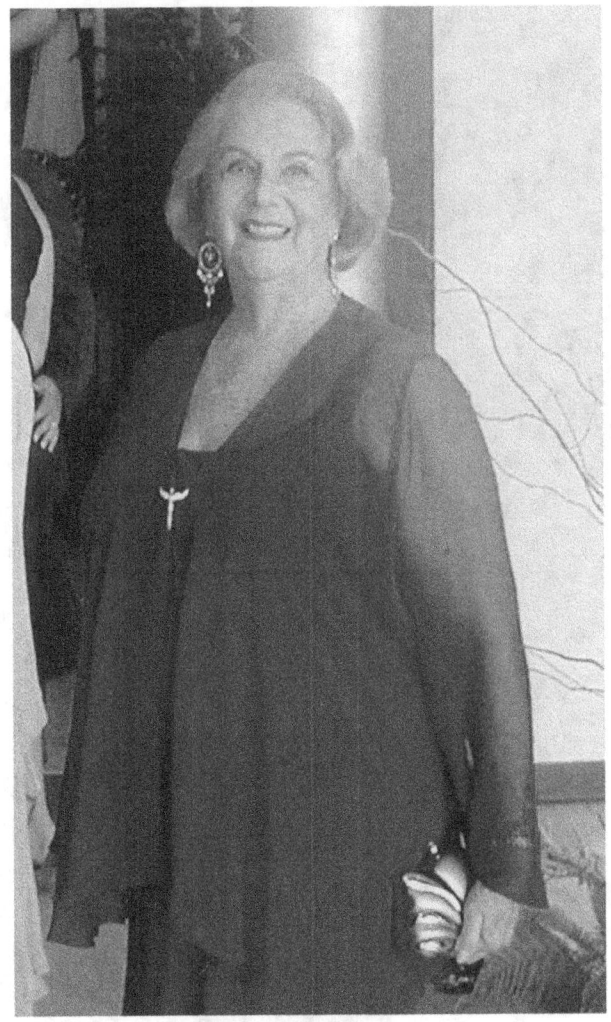

Martha looking positively regal at 82

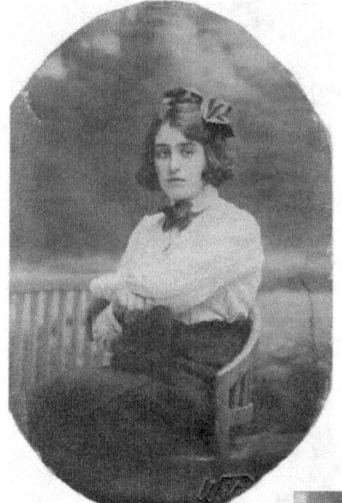

Martha's mother, Elvira,
aged 18

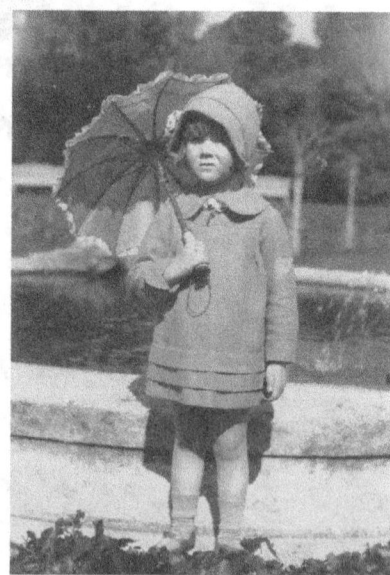

Young Martha

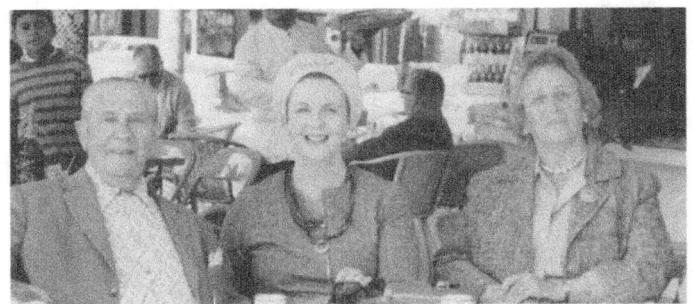

Martha and her parents

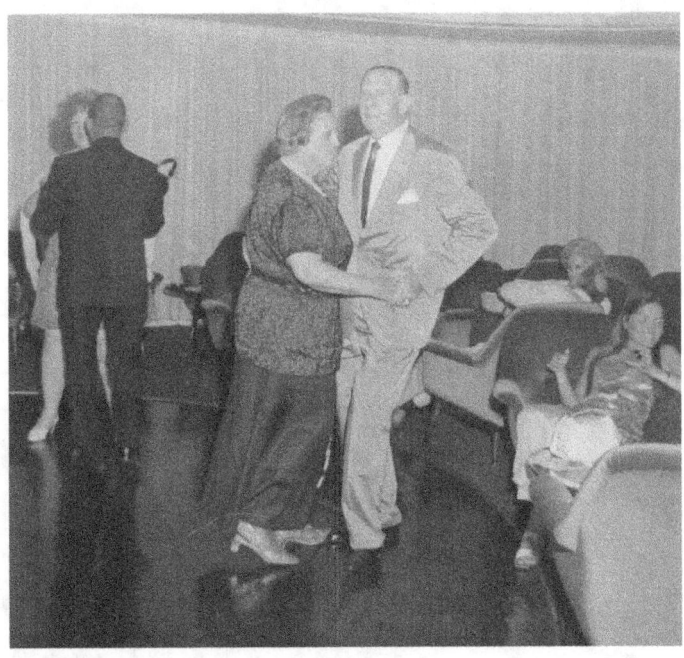

Martha's parents - still dancing the Tango in their 70s

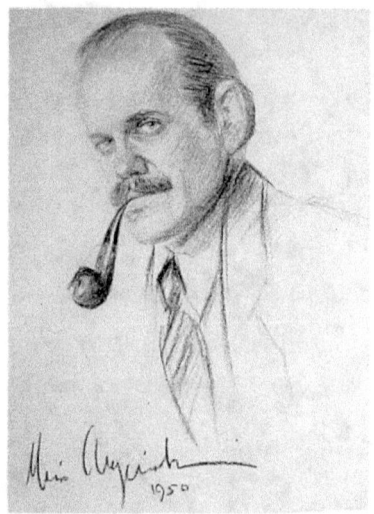

A treasured charcoal drawing of
Martha's husband, Alberto

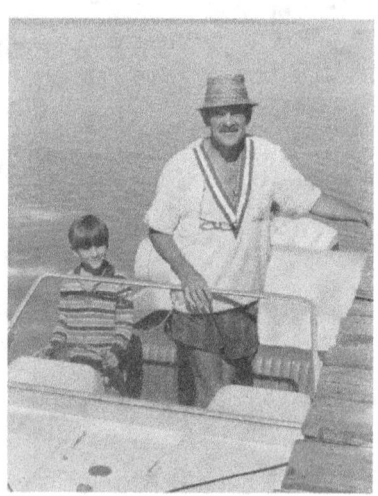

Rodrigo with his father

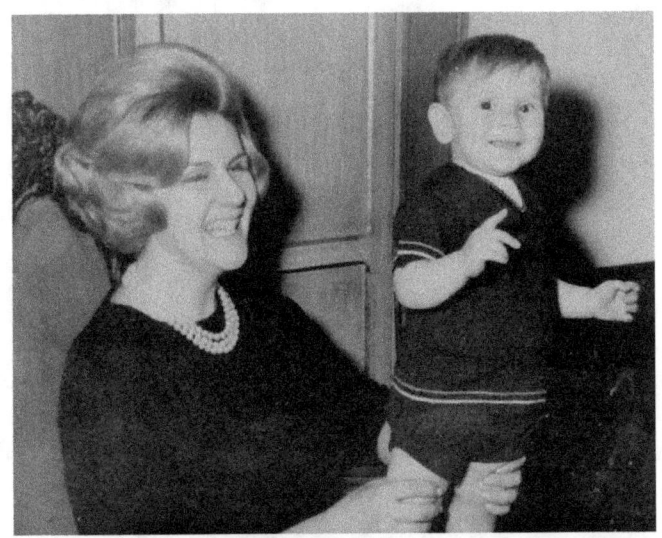

Martha with Rodrigo

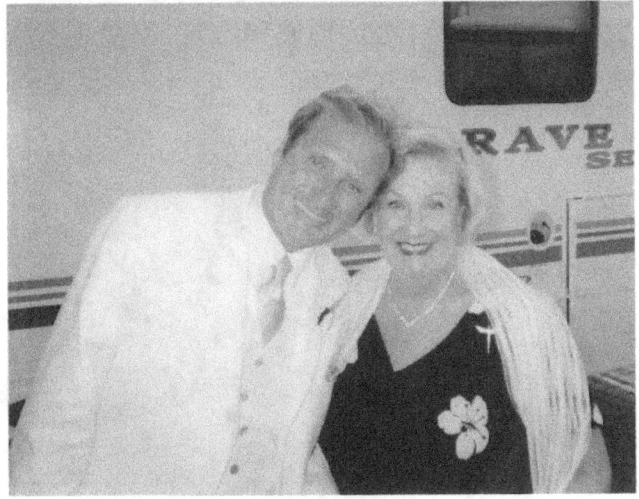

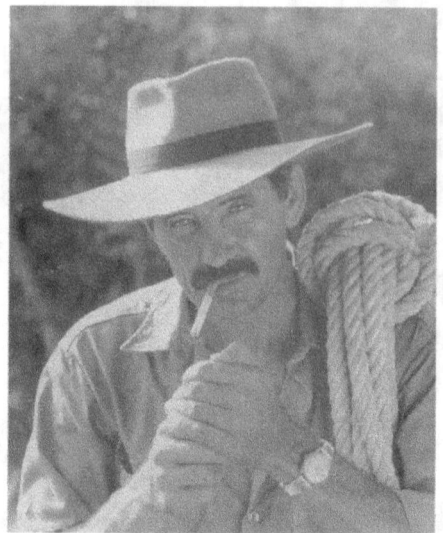

Carlos as the Latin American Marlboro Man

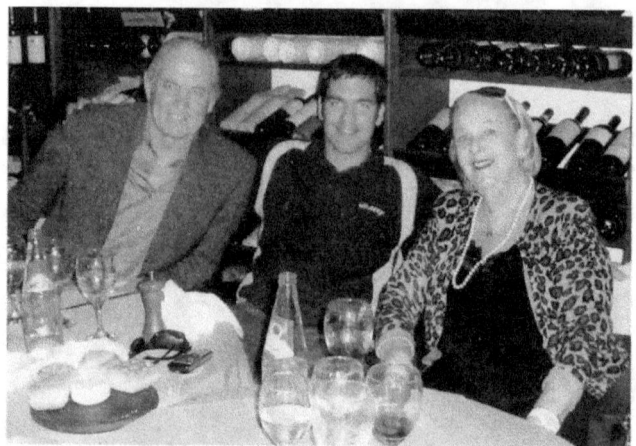

Martha with Carlos and his son, Francisco

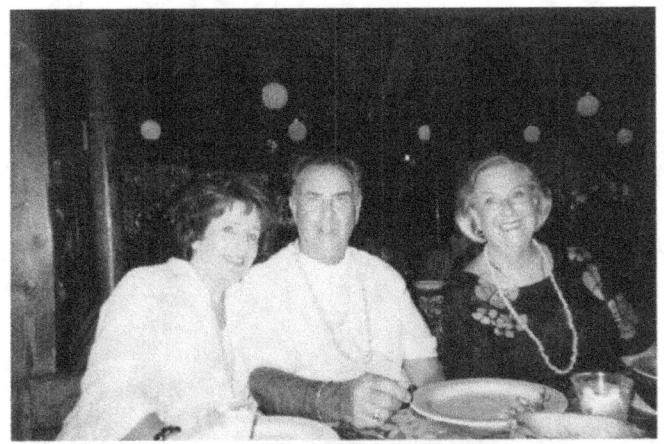

Martha with her brother Hugo and his wife, Norah

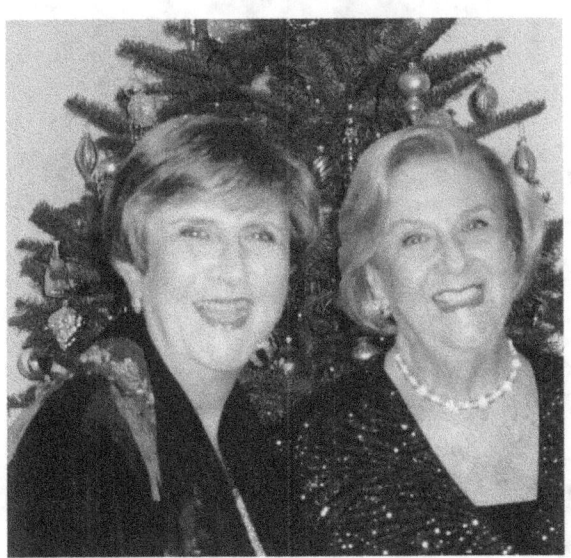

Devoted sisters, Susana and Martha

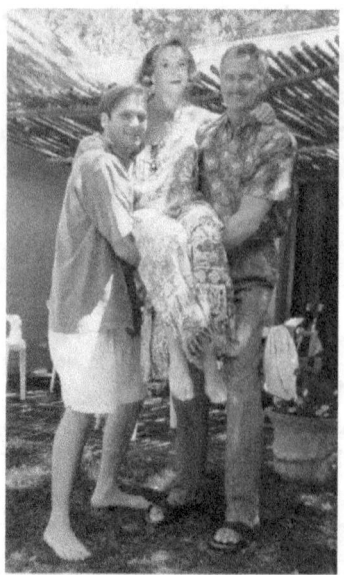

Martha with her sons Rodrigo (left) and Carlos

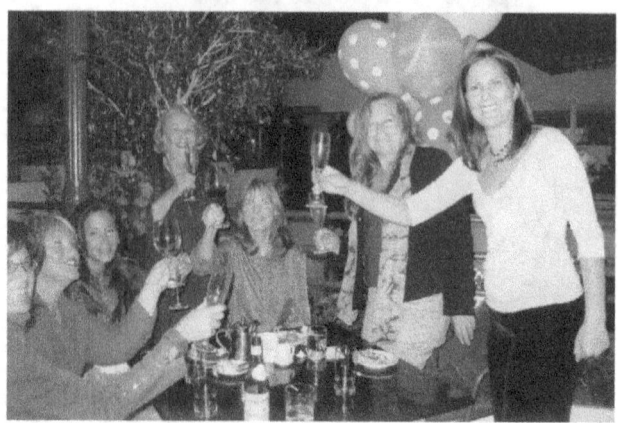

Stay Young Revolutionaries toast Martha and the revolution!

4

TO BE OR NOT TO BE

A national hero Argentina shares with several other South American countries (who also liberated them from Spanish rule) is General Don Jose de San Martin. As children in school, we heard about him all the time in history and music, singing songs to him. Every time a teacher or the principal gave a speech, his picture presided over the classroom. A bronze statue of him on a horse is in the main park or plaza of every major town in Argentina.

I felt great respect for him as a founding father, but could never understand his message until recently. I was trying to think of an inspirational phrase for a book I was writing and I suddenly realized it was basically the same thing General José de San Martín used to motivate his troops, "You will be what you have to be, otherwise you will be nothing."

The light turned on for me. He was saying that unless you

become what you're destined to be, your life will be void of meaning. This is close to how I feel when I'm trying to inspire people to be what they dream of being. To go against prejudices and limitations, against obsolete belief systems and boundaries, to make their own choices, to live a life full of meaning and purpose. Thank you, General. It took me a while, but that seed you planted so long ago is now bringing light to my consciousness.

It is around this concept that I saw my path taking form and becoming a passion. I want to create tools for people to feel good about themselves, feel confident, be able to love and help others because they had started to like and love themselves first.

My small contribution to that goal of higher self esteem and realization was to create a better image, a younger presence, a more beautiful and attractive look. Instead of just preaching concepts, I was — and still am — hands-on, transforming faces and bodies into their better-looking, healthier selves. My thinking is: Healthy, attractive people are happier. Happier people make a better world.

So join the revolution and let's change the world. To be or not to be? You can be. I can be. Everyone can be.

5

THE TABLE METAPHOR

If we could compare our lives to a dining room table, what would you like to see on yours? Imagine you can choose what the table can display. How rich and attractive would you make it?

Over the years, I have visualized my table in many different ways, sometimes even holding terrible combinations of things. A good lesson was to learn how to live in the present. But of something I was always sure: the four legs had to be the same length. Otherwise the table would tilt and all the good stuff would end up on the floor.

The four legs that support the table of our life are the four aspects that form our existence: mental, emotional, physical and spiritual. Having those legs carefully balanced and permanently considered, makes for a stable and satisfying life.

It may be that sometimes one or more of the legs are being neglected and lacking attention. Then the quality of life is jeopardized. A quick re-assessment of values is needed and the table can again be a happy and healthy one.

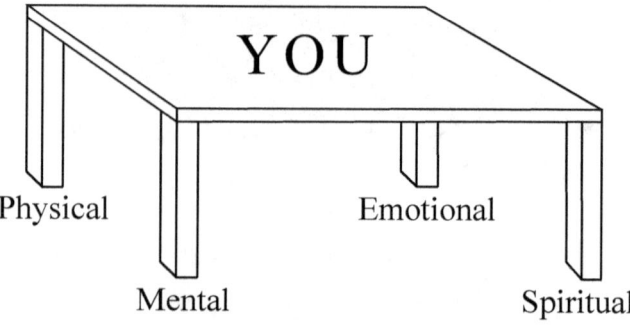

Stay Young Revolutionaries (SYRs) have to pay attention to their table legs and reinforce the ones that need more support.

THE PHYSICAL ASPECT

What you eat and drink

Your sleeping habits

How you release physical stress

The amount of exercise you do

How you look

How you dress

Your medical advisors

THE MENTAL ASPECT

Keep your mind active by learning about new things and ideas

Keep your mind exercised by embracing new technologies

Communicate with younger people

Be creative – make things or sing, act, dance, paint, draw or write

Stress – learn ways to overcome anxiety

Be accepting of others and yourself

THE EMOTIONAL ASPECT

Do things you enjoy – vacations, entertainment, fun activities and relationships

Connect regularly with people you love or like

Find ways to release emotional stress

Have love and passion in your life

Enjoy your work

Acknowledge your dreams and desires

Acknowledge and understand your fears

THE SPIRITUAL ASPECT

Understand how life, death and the universe work for you

Be present. Concentrate on the now, not the past or the future

Be clear regarding your religious beliefs and spiritual beliefs, and be at peace with them

6

NOURISHING THE BODY

I use a lot of royal jelly in my cosmetic products because it's the most concentrated nourishment in nature and it is easily absorbed by the skin. I also listen to music. It nourishes my soul.

Louis Armstrong inspires me. "When the Saints Go Marching In" is the ringtone on my cell phone. Every time I answer the phone, the rhythm puts me in a good mood.

The entire universe functions according to rhythm. We obey laws of nature. In the field of nutrition, circadian rhythms determine that the same foods eaten at different times of the day provide different nutritional values.

That cheese omelet you like so much will nourish you differently if you eat it at 10am or 10pm because your metabolism is different. You should eat it in the morning.

You should never eat a big meal after 6pm unless you're planning on making love all night. But this book isn't just about me saying cute things. I am offering you strategies and technologies to live long and well.

It's normal to have high and low energy at different times throughout the day and you are just following natural cycles. When you feel the need for a shot in the arm that a strong double espresso will give you, it's because you are on a down cycle.

Instead of artificially stimulating your central nervous system with caffeine, which will soon fade and send you back to the coffee line with the rest of the cranky crowd, try falling in love with trail mix.

I make my own combination of nuts, seeds, dried fruits and dried yogurt, and keep some handy in the car. You can easily buy trail mix ready made. If I get hungry or tired while driving, I can replenish my energy with something healthy.

A handful of trail mix mid-morning or mid-afternoon helps keep my energy balanced. If trail mix doesn't sound appealing, you can create your own equivalent using easily absorbed protein like hummus or edamame beans.

And to drink? How about a nice steaming cup of herbal tea with a spoonful of honey? In sophisticated places, they offer lattes made with herbal teas. Try one. Shake it up.

Many people don't realize that there are always options. I promise you that when you pluck up the courage to step outside your comfort zone and break old habits and patterns, you will feel great.

I'm always looking to try something new. It requires research and effort, but it's exhilarating.

What comes next is a kind of grocery list of all the things you need to consider and keep track of for the best possible results if you want to look and feel younger and be healthy.

We are looking to keep the physical, mental, emotional and spiritual worlds in balance. All of them are equally important and neglecting any area will bring instability and suffering into your life. Not a good way to go if you want to stay young.

Beautify & Tone

The Non-Invasive Face Lift

The procedure that brought me wide recognition is the non-invasive facelift. It really works. And here's how.

The health of all cells is based on cellular energy. When this energy diminishes, cells become weaker and the body's organs suffer the consequences, like premature aging and illness. Maintaining the right amount and kind of energy at the cellular level is vitally important in retaining youthfulness.

Restorative effects start at the atomic level. We know atoms make up the cells, which make up the tissues, which make up the organs, which make up entire systems like our human body.

My Stay Young System works by restoring the right kind and right amount of energy to the skin, connective tissues and muscles of the face and neck. It revitalizes skin cells with a gentle, low-level, bio-identical galvanic nano-current, precisely calibrated to activate the natural energy in your skin.

It's applied using hand-held electrodes. The system is preprogrammed to adjust to the different areas of the face and neck, and re-energizes tissue by strengthening cells so the aging process is modified and the skin can stay young for longer.

Just like your body, your face needs an exercise program. This technology stimulates facial muscles to exercise themselves, helping the skin to maintain its tone and youthful glow for years to come. It feels like a gentle massage, but the result is immediate and dramatic after each twenty-five-minute treatment as collagen production and elasticity is increased.

Faces look visibly smoother, radiant and rejuvenated. To establish strong muscle memory, I recommend a series of ten to fifteen weekly treatments followed by a monthly maintenance program.

By the time I was in my eighties, I had been using such systems for more than twenty years. They had been simplified from plugging into a wall outlet to being battery operated, but practitioners and estheticians found the old machines cumbersome and complicated. I developed a simpler system that automatically incorporated the correct current for each area of the face and neck.

I found an electronic engineer who understood my concept and together we created a machine with pre-established settings. I believe my system is the only one where you have to press just one button and everything is pre-set.

My first machine for use in salons was effective but bulky. Desktop computers had become laptops, so I thought, *maybe we can do the same with my machine.*

The portable, laptop version of my machine, "The Stay Young System," is also battery powered, with protocols for personal and professional use. There's a clear and easy-to-understand step-by-step guide I wrote myself.

The price is affordable and lasts a lifetime. If you have your own machine, you have the freedom to have two or three shorter sessions a week where you can focus on problem areas.

There are other, cheaper machines out there, but they don't get the same results as mine because the combination of settings is not correct. They are toys compared with mine.

Most of my regular clients have bought one, but still come in for a monthly maintenance session with me or one of my estheticians so they get a good zapping. It's lovely to lie on a table as a beauty therapist massages your face rather than do it yourself all the time. It's important to be pampered every once in a while.

The system isn't recommended for pregnant women or if you have epilepsy or heart problems. Certainly not if you have metal implants in your face, neck or head.

People who have mercury fillings in their teeth have occasionally reported a metallic taste during the procedure, but they are not incompatible. I've never had any complaints, and my clients look and feel amazing.

I want to share my invention with as many people as possible because it saves them having to do more invasive treatments – and you know how I feel about plastic surgery. That's why I called it The Non-Invasive Face Lift. There are no cuts, no injections, no fillers. There is nothing artificial about it, just replacing the electrical energy to the cells.

I have different parts of the system manufactured around the world and they are assembled in the United States. I won't go into too much detail, as that is part of my business secret that keeps me in control of what I'm making.

A crucial aspect of letting people have their own machine is to give them the correct training and certification so they use the system correctly. I always require that they complete a brief training program with me or one of my specialists and that's included in the price.

My Non-Invasive Face Lift using bio-identical nano-current reduces wrinkles and lines, improves skin health, moisturizes, and revitalizes. There is no downside.

An especially popular benefit of the system is that it also helps plump up the lips. It's barely noticeable, but clients find their lipstick no longer "bleeds" like it used to. They can't put their finger on what's changed, but they know they look younger and more attractive, with lips better defined and more "juicy."

The husband of one of my regular clients came to see me for a session. When he left, he said, "Thank you for making my wife's lips more kissable." I said, "You're welcome. Now yours will be too."

5 Steps Daily Program

If you want to have great skin, you must have a beauty

routine every day of your life. To make skin look and feel its best, we need to cleanse, moisturize, protect, exfoliate and nourish. Those are the five steps. All beauty experts agree on that.

However, after almost seventy years' experience as a beauty therapist and having been married to a cosmetic chemist, I am confident my five-step skincare range is as effective as any.

What you use on your skin on a daily basis is what makes the real difference. I don't think there are any magical ingredients or one product that can do many things. That's why I call mine a synergistic skincare program. This means that all the ingredients in my products work in combination, and are more effective when used together.

Working as a team, Alberto Iglesias and I created a collection of plant-based products with added minerals and proteins. It's a simple system where using the correct combination produces an optimum result that supports the skin's five basic needs in order to be balanced and radiant. You need the synergy of products working in combination.

Over the years, my 5 Steps Daily Program has evolved to include the best modern ingredients and combinations available – always the best ingredients. This is an easy, affordable, balanced and pleasant program my clients can use at home. I call it their homework. Steps One and Two are performed in the morning; Steps Three, Four and Five in the evening.

Of course, you don't *have* to use my skincare range. You can create your own five steps with your favorite products as long as those five essential needs of the skin are being covered.

Hair

While I believe that beautiful, firm and clear skin is the most important aspect to looking as youthful as possible (looking so great that people gasp "wow" when they hear how old you are), we need to pay attention to all areas, because we are the sum of all our parts.

Other aspects of grooming play a big part in our overall beauty regimen and although it would take a separate book to do them justice, I want to mention them here. Let's start at the top and work down.

There are two aspects to good hair: the health aspect and the fashion aspect. As you age, the look and consistency of your hair plays a big part in how people perceive your age. I am lucky in that department.

My hairdresser says, "I don't even have to tease your hair, there is so much of it." But I know not every ninety-year-old has good hair. It has to do with how they took care of themselves from day one – how healthily we eat, what vitamins we take, and how we style and color our hair.

Of course, there are a few older women who look spectacular with grey or white hair. But you have to trust me on this: grey hair is aging. Men can look distinguished with grey hair, but we just look like our mothers. Grey hair makes us look at least twenty years older.

Unless you know very well what you are doing, I would always recommend having a professional hairdresser color and cut your hair. Some hair responds better to color than others. It depends on the health and strength of the root follicle and shaft.

My hair started to go grey when I was twenty-five. Not all over, but too many to ignore. I have colored my hair every four to five weeks ever since. It's healthy and grows fast, so my grey roots appear mercilessly.

It can be really dangerous to color your hair yourself. I've seen some major disasters. At the very least, home-colored hair tends to lose its shine. If you're not as good as a professional, please don't mess with your hair yourself.

As a good revolutionary should do, I change my hair color every few months. For a long time, I was different tones of blonde. I like to shake it up. Right now, I have a dark base on my roots with highlights. It needs to be the right contrast between the base and the highlights and it looks younger.

Good quality products are also important when coloring your hair or you will destroy the keratin, a key structural component in skin, hair and nails. The healthier your hair, the quicker and thicker it grows. A diet rich in calcium, vitamins and minerals is vital for good hair, skin, nails, bones and teeth.

It's not just harsh chemicals in coloring products that cause harm. Curling and straightening irons can cause enormous damage when they are used incorrectly or overused.

A good haircut is also important. That's where the fashion aspect comes in.

Everyone used to choose a cut that best suited their face. The most beautiful, becoming and flattering facial shape was always considered to be oval. These days, many people want to look like their favorite celebrity even if they have square, rectangular or round faces.

A great cutter and stylist can make anything work. A layered cut will soften a square-shaped face. A rectangular face needs a longer, layered cut. But there are no rules these days. I've seen blue, green and pink hair.

It takes a true artist, however, to create a hairstyle that looks natural but still amazing. That's why some stylists become famous for their skills and command high fees.

Eyebrows

Eyebrows are so important. They frame and shape the face and give a distinctive look. If your eyebrows aren't well shaped or are neglected, you might be losing a big part of your attraction.

If you have very little hair or your eyebrows have no definition, there are excellent permanent make-up artists who can fake your eyebrows and make them look natural and beautiful with a nice arching that will frame your eyes to make you look a lot more interesting.

As you would take great care to choose a good hairdresser, someone advising you about permanent make-up should also come highly recommended.

Facial hair

A woman was complaining to her therapist that she couldn't find the right partner. The therapist said, "Maybe you should do something about your moustache?"

Too much facial hair can be a major problem for some women and often plucking just isn't enough. If you don't take care of it, you will look like a woman who doesn't care how they look.

Bleaching alone doesn't take the hair off, so you might need to try waxing. There are chemical creams that will remove it, but, again, go to an expert.

Lasers remove unwanted hair permanently, but they are only effective on dark hairs and whiskers, not grey or white.

Another type of facial hair that doesn't look attractive is fuzz. After certain hormonal changes, a fluff appears on the side of the face that is easy to wax away and you don't have to do it very often. A waxing every four months should keep it at bay and it doesn't grow back like a beard. It remains fluff. I specialize in the Non Invasive Face Lift, but when my clients need a little help in other departments I have no problem in doing it.

Make-up

For everyday use, keep make-up simple. Nowadays, there are good tinted moisturizers that give the skin protection and color at the same time.

Well-defined eyebrows, a good lipstick and a fine line on the upper eyelid are all you need to look good. If you like to have long lashes, there are products that make them grow and they can look great with a little mascara. You can also tint the eyelashes if they're too light.

More elaborate make-up needs practice. Imagine your face is a canvas and experiment with different colors and looks. There's no harm in it as it can be easily removed.

Fashion changes constantly and so does your face and mood. Make-up is something to have fun with. Find a look you're comfortable with and suits you.

Hands and feet

Soap can be extremely harsh and eliminates the skin's natural oils, so use a light moisturizer on your hands every time you wash them. Keep some hand cream in the kitchen to use every time you wash your hands after cooking.

Moisturize your feet daily as well, or hard skin will develop on the soles. You can do it after your shower with a good body lotion.

Keep your fingernails and toenails clean and shaped. Nail lacquer adds the finishing touch to good grooming. A good manicurist and pedicurist can be your best friend.

Teeth

Make sure your chewing apparatus is in the best possible shape. As you age, if you're teeth aren't in good condition then you don't chew well or chew properly. That affects not only your nutrition but the look of your teeth.

Regular check-ups and cleanings are vital. I believe strongly that dental work is a wise investment to keep everything in your mouth as healthy as possible. Bad teeth are not only unhealthy but most unattractive.

Smiling

Many wrinkles around the eyes are produced by smiling There's a right way and a wrong way to smile. When most people smile, they squint. Do that too much and you will get a lot of wrinkles.

Try to smile without squinting. It's a technique that takes practice, but it works. Look in the mirror. Smile. Keep your eyes open but don't squint. Smiling this way has saved me from many wrinkles around my eyes.

When I had my beauty school, every six months I had to give diplomas to hundreds of girls and everyone of them wanted a photograph with me. I had to develop a technique to keep my eyes open and not squint when I smiled for those photos. Just try it.

Weight

One terrible fact of life is that it's far more difficult to lose extra weight as we grow older. But there's a big difference between being slightly overweight and obese. Inches are more important than pounds, in my opinion.

The sensible thing to do is reduce your portions, cut down your sugar and fat intakes. Keep your mouth shut, exercise and eat real food!

This is a delicate issue. Some people become obsessed with their weight and like everything that becomes an obsession, it doesn't help your life.

If you're seriously concerned about your weight, consult a nutritionist who can recommend the right diet for your lifestyle and body shape. But avoid crash diets at all costs and, most importantly, don't be obsessed by it.

To understand how the storage of fat works in our bodies, SYRs need to understand how insulin works and to make it your friend.

Insulin is a hormone produced by the pancreas that regulates the level of glucose, a simple sugar that provides energy, in the blood. The human body requires a steady amount of glucose throughout the day, which comes from the foods we eat.

When we go for a blood test, one of the things doctors pay most attention to is how much sugar we have in our blood. Too much sugar in our blood is poison, with terrible consequences on our health.

If the pancreas stops producing the correct amount of

insulin, you become diabetic and have to inject yourself with insulin to regulate the levels.

We don't have to be a diabetic to have a tendency to gain weight, because the sugar we eat it is stored as fat on our hips, stomach or wherever else the body stores extra fat deposits.

So as well as counting calories in and out, we need to avoid having too much sugar in the bloodstream and ensure our insulin-making mechanism is functioning properly.

Excess sugar in the bloodstream makes it harder to burn fat, even with exercise. We can all benefit from avoiding foods that have high sugar content, such as all the starches and sweets, and even some fruits. That includes delicious things like potatoes, bread and rice. Eat more protein and less sugary fruits like grapes, apples and pears.

Today I had a lunch rich in protein after my water aerobics class. I ate a small salad, some scrambled eggs and a piece of broiled chicken breast – nothing that could be transformed into fat. A high-protein diet also gives you more energy.

There are many good diets out there and I don't want to

compete with them, but insulin production is an essential mechanism that one has to understand. Because as we grow older, our metabolism slows down and we burn even fewer calories. So we have to eliminate (certainly avoid) foods that turn easily into fat.

Detoxify

An SYR should not smoke. When you smoke cigarettes, you put deadly nicotine in your system that deprives the skin and body of vital oxygen. No wonder women who smoke have a sallow complexion, wrinkles, premature sagging and lifeless-looking eyes. We also know that smoking greatly increases the risk of heart disease and lung cancer.

I smoked for about four years between eighteen and twenty-two, and I got so sick I had to stop just to survive. It was incredibly difficult to stop because, like any addiction, it controls you. That's what big tobacco companies are after, to enslave people.

I think it's wonderful that smoking is considered almost a crime in many of our cities. And rightly so, because it's poisoning every cell in your body and those of the people unlucky enough to be around you who inhale your second-hand smoke.

With alcohol it's a question of quantity. In France, where most people have a couple of glasses of red wine every day, it's an amount that's good for the circulation. It's another story when you drink hard liquor and too much of it.

I never felt a need to take recreational drugs. I'm not an expert, but I certainly wouldn't recommend them. In the same way, I suggest people take the least prescription drugs as possible. People get addicted to those too. They affect metabolism and psychology. Lives are changed and not for the better.

I often wonder why they're called recreational drugs. How can something be called recreational when it's killing you? Merchants will always invent a good excuse to sell their poisons. You don't have to believe them.

Energize

Massage and mobility

Everything that stimulates circulation is helpful in keeping us young. The most important is regular exercise. Whether it's yoga, Zumba or walking, find something you enjoy and get moving. I'm also a great believer in massage which has existed since ancient times. Deep tissue Swedish massage is especially effective and popular in the West.

A massage therapist works on muscles to stimulate blood circulation and send nutrients to all parts of the body so you don't feel sluggish. Massage works and you feel great afterwards. In combination with regular exercise, massage will help keep your muscles toned and firm, your spine flexible and your joints lubricated.

Supplements

We are living in a society where we're expected to take a lot of medications after a certain age. Maybe I'm being difficult, but I refuse to contribute to the financial health of any pharmaceutical conglomerate. I'd rather take supplements. If you take enough of the right supplements, you probably won't be taking so many medications, and only when you're sick.

In my experience, there are basic supplements everyone should take because our food is usually so over-processed it doesn't always provide enough of them. And those are vitamins and minerals. When you're not getting enough essential vitamins and minerals, you reduce your chances for a good performance and cheat yourself out of your potential.

There are other supplements that constitute a support system for your entire life. As important as the mind and soul are, they cannot manifest properly if the organs through which they perform are not functioning at optimum levels. If your brain is not healthy, your mind is diminished. If your nervous system is deprived of its essential nutrients your emotions will be distorted. At this level, we have to put emphasis on the body because the body is the connector.

Many illnesses can be prevented by choosing to eat well and by taking the right supplements. Several aspects of our performance in life can be enhanced by utilizing the right supplements.

While there are recommended daily allowances for vitamins and minerals, everyone is different and you have to do your own research, taking note of how you feel and what you would like to elevate in your performance.

As well as a daily multi-vitamin and mineral supplement, I take a daily dose of effective antioxidants that help with many of the symptoms of premature aging and can be found among the most reliable supplement brands.

Firstly, let me remind you what free radicals do to your system: they attack the membranes of your cells so those cells start to function poorly and even die. The body has a defence system of antioxidants that can safely interact with free radicals before vital molecules are damaged. If these molecules are compromised, it sets off a process of disease and accelerated aging. So antioxidants help your system fight free radicals.

My favorite antioxidant is grape seed extract, for its great ability to fight the free radicals that produce erosion and dysfunction in our bodies.

Grape seed extract helps me to control my carpal tunnel syndrome, arthritis and mental fatigue. I have been taking it for nearly twenty-five years and it's one of the elements I credit for my longevity.

Before I started taking grape seed extract regularly at age sixty-five I was tired when I finished my week's work. In our profession, we usually work Saturdays, so when I was finishing at 5.30pm, I had no stamina to go to parties or the movies or do anything else but go home and crash. My weekends began on Sundays when I usually drove for two hours to enjoy some time with my sister at our weekend home in the desert.

Once I started to take grape seed extract, I had the energy to make the two-hour drive after work on Saturdays. I have no doubt that it was adding that supplement to my daily routine that gave me the resilience I was looking for to start the weekend sooner and wake up the next morning already there.

I slowly increased my dose of grape seed extract from 50 milligrams to 300 milligrams a day, every day. If I stop taking it for a couple of days, the pain returns to my wrists. But when I resume, I am pain-free and able to perform dozens of facial treatments.

Other useful supplements are Omega 3, healthy fatty acids that promote healthy joints and Evening Primrose Oil that's used in alternative medicine as an aid in treating heart disease, high cholesterol, circulation problems, endometriosis, breast pain, some symptoms of menopause, eczema, psoriasis, and osteoporosis.

Vitamin C is also an antioxidant and enhances the immune system so you can be better prepared to fight common illnesses. To help your skin internally, vitamin E is highly recommended, and other supplements like calcium citrate with vitamin D help prevent osteoporosis.

If you have severe symptoms and not just feeling under par, consult your physician or your natural medicine consultant for more detailed supplementation advice.

Relax

There are many reasons why we experience low energy, but the worse one is probably the stress of everyday living. Learning to relax will help keep your energy at the right level. I know it's hard to relax in these frenetic times, but here are some tips on how I do it and have done through the most active years of my life. I've seen many friends, relatives and clients benefit from following these tips to cope with stressful situations, avoid feeling drained and even alleviate depression.

When people ask me, "How do you keep your energy all day long?" I reply, "I take naps." I also call them mini-breaks. So when I feel tired, I take a short nap – just five or ten minutes of letting go. Sometimes I listen to a relaxation tape for half an hour and then I feel like a new person. My quality of life is severely compromised when I am over-tired.

Exercising can also be relaxing. So can playing a sport. Even plain playing and having fun can relax you. Meditation is extremely relaxing. Taking short breaks at work can help. Find your recipe for relaxation to make sure you are not letting down your mental and physical stamina.

I have a built-in alarm clock that rings loudly when I need to rest. *Ring! Ring! Martha, it's time to relax!*

The important thing is to know instinctively when you need to recharge your batteries. Listen to your body. Pay attention to your energy levels instead of ignoring the signals sent by your mind and body.

Set up the alarm clock that works for you. *Ring! Ring! Time to relax!*

If you ignore the ring too many times, you pay the consequences. Instead of accumulating stress all day, you can choose to accumulate relaxation. Then you can live with just one apple martini at the end of the day instead of three.

Some people think they're relaxing, but they aren't. Changing your routine isn't always enough. I have a great co-worker whose idea of relaxing is to take a day off work, then she stays at home and deals with all the problems of the people around her: her son, niece, roommate and her cat. Of course, when she comes back to work from a day of "relaxation" she has deep, dark circles under her eyes and doesn't look relaxed at all.

My idea of relaxation is to disconnect from all sources of stress. That allows me to bounce back and face whatever challenge comes my way.

There is a science to staying young and the lesson on how to relax correctly is a vitally important one. You will find more recommendations on how to keep your energy in balance when we talk about foods that help prevent fatigue, instead of stimulating your performance with a fleeting burst of false well-being from caffeine or alcohol.

"The Dog's Corner" is one of my favorite short stories by my late husband, Alberto Iglesias. Although Alberto has passed away, he is still part of my entourage, according to my psychic. This story is about the importance of having your own place, a corner where you can go and lick your wounds and regroup – a little corner of the world where you are protected, and feels like yours and yours alone. It doesn't have to be an elaborate place. Even a favorite chair in your office or recliner at home can be your refuge.

In 1965, I attended a congress in Brussels for women entrepreneurs. It was sponsored by Queen Fabiola of Belgium, a Spanish aristocrat who married King Baudouin and was always supportive of women's issues. When I was introduced to Her Majesty at the opening ceremony, I handed her a book I brought from Argentina that portrayed the life of the gauchos and was like a bible in my country.

The Queen thanked me very much for the present, but never touched it with her own hands. I had to place it in the hands of an aide. Then she looked at me warmly and said, "Whenever I want to relax, I close my eyes and think of Bariloche."

That remark touched me deeply (the proof is that I have remembered it for forty years) because I, too, love the beautiful lakes and mountains of Bariloche in Southern Argentina, where the royal couple vacationed every summer.

I share this anecdote with you so if you don't have a dog's corner of your own, you can close your eyes and imagine one. If The Queen of Belgium can do it, you and I can do it too.

MARTHA WEINSTEIN

7

NOURISHING THE MIND

As well as feeding our body, we must feed the mind. When it comes to nourishing the mind, there is one rule: keep feeding it new information. Learn something new – a skill, another language, or a game. Anything that really challenges the mind keeps it flexible and interested. Nourishing the mind should be practiced throughout life. It doesn't matter how old you are, you need to feed your mind fresh and exciting information.

At seventy-nine, I started learning to paint with watercolors. I took an educational tour with a group of travelers to a beautiful spot in Georgia, where we had painting lessons. I really felt I was challenging my mind and creativity because I had access to a different perception, combining colors and shapes. It really felt wonderful. And then, at eighty-one, I suddenly had this urge to learn how to make custom jewelry. Never neglect your urges. I followed mine by finding an inspiring instructor who gave wonderful classes.

Now I have a table at home that is my workshop. Half of it is for water color painting and the other half is for making jewelry. Whenever I have time or feel inspired, I just go to one of the sides of the table and do something with either activity. It's a lot of fun.

A few years ago, my son Rodrigo had just returned from Costa Rica and bought me a beautiful hematite and quartz necklace. I loved it, but when I put it on I could not find earrings to go with it. So I sat at the jewelry end of the table, found the right stones and made a pair.

Jewelry making enriches my mind and soul and made my son laugh. I was shaking my head, making my earrings dance. We were both looking in the mirror and he said, "Are you really eighty-three?"

Go ahead, have some fun. Nourish yourself. I learned about the concept of having fun from my friend, Matilde. She is a psychotherapist and concentrates all her work and efforts on protecting, healing and helping the inner child.

I think this is such an important area to consider, for people to recognize and nourish their inner child. If you can keep yourself childlike, you will always be open to surprises and the new wonders that fill the universe. It makes everything so much brighter, so much more appealing and provides little moments of fun during the seriousness of the day.

How about choosing to live your life with your inner child wanting to peek out and be part of what's going on? A child always wants to be part of events. Remember when you were a child? You are still one inside. Keep your inner child close to the surface. Make sure you always let it come out to play.

New technologies

I have made many new friends at the water aerobics class I attend three times a week. We are aged between eighteen and eighty-nine (me). They always tease me that I am the only eighty-nine-year-old they know who uses a smart phone and iPad when their relatives don't even know how to find the right buttons.

It makes my classmates laugh that I know how to use new technologies and the buzzwords for them, when I talk about the optimization of my website, how to make a website active and bring traffic to it, but it also keeps my business alive. Embracing new technology is an excellent way to get your brain jogging.

Nowadays, forms of advertising and connecting with people is mostly through the Internet. The old advertising approaches no longer work. Newspapers and magazines are disappearing and the only place people are really looking at for information is the Internet. So if you don't keep up with the times, you're completely out of the game. And I don't want to be out of the game.

My concept of staying young involves understanding blogs, Facebook, Twitter – all the sites where you connect with people. And if you want to maintain contact with your grandchildren, you must be able to text.

I've mentioned before how the thousands of women I educated in Argentina are re-connecting with me after all these years via Facebook, thanking me for helping them create a career that enabled them to educate their children. If I wasn't on Facebook, I wouldn't have been contacted all these years later by former students who say, "I thank you very much for being so bold in those days and telling women that they should take care of themselves, be independent, feel confident, create their own sources of income and be an example to their children. Not only because they were beautiful and hardworking, but because they were looking into the future with a spirit of conquest. You wanted to conquer a new way of behaving, thinking and enjoying life, and you did."

Don't rush to be ready

Like fine wine in a bottle, some ideas need to mature in your brain until they age to perfection. Don't be frustrated about change taking too long to happen. Once you've set your intention, things will start changing at any time if it's what you really want.

One of my favorite authors, Harry Bernstein, began writing his riveting memoir, *The Invisible Wall*, at ninety-six. He said, "If I had not lived until I was ninety, I would not have been able to write this book. Ten years ago, I wasn't ready. God only knows what great potential lurks in other people if you could only keep them alive well into their nineties."

That applies to me too. I wasn't ready to start a revolution ten years ago. I am now eighty-nine and still don't feel old. If you don't believe me, come to my salon and watch me. I am in the business of making people feel good about themselves.

Nowadays, I work in my small day spa that specializes in "stay young" programs for all ages. It's a cliché to say that prevention is the best medicine, but I believe it.

My staff and I also believe there are many ways to slow down the ravages of time and restore beauty to a face and a body without using invasive procedures. I have developed most of my best programs in the last twelve years. I have done my best work in my seventies.

Being productive makes me extremely happy. I have no problem working many hours a day. Seeing people flourish after one of my treatments inspires me to keep going. They act differently and see that doing something for themselves brings the energy of renewal. They look better, so they feel better. My greatest reward is when my clients look in the mirror after one of my facial treatments and say, "I love it."

I don't expect the entire world to come to my salon to have treatments with me (that actually might age me a bit), but I want to share what you can accomplish for yourselves, for your own good and for humankind, as you grow into the person you are meant to be.

Tell me right now, what are you doing to feel better about yourself?

The energy from renewal can come from many different sources. I have a friend who takes a class once a week to improve her conversational French. From this one-hour "indulgence" she is a changed person. Every morning she listens to her tapes and feels proud of the progress she is making. From that simple experience, she gets so much pleasure and gratification. This is what I want for you: to find an "indulgence" that is really a necessity.

Waiting to reach maturity doesn't mean you haven't accomplished many valuable things in life. The point is that certain things you might have stored in your mind will not reach the surface until you are ready. And that may take time.

Don't abandon hope that great new projects won't happen for you. They can happen any time. Don't close the door on possible accomplishments that are at the core of your heart's desire. It's never too late.

Have you given up before really giving yourself a chance? Seeds planted long ago in your subconscious are waiting to become flowers of great beauty. Just keep yourself receptive as the soil nurtures those seeds of creativity to bloom.

Don't let your "soil" get contaminated by the general assumption that after a certain age you cannot be creative. Don't let anything or anyone stop you.

My friend Alex retired twenty years ago, stayed at home for a week and quickly un-retired. He has been happily employed since then. He gets up, goes to the gym and then goes to work at the same car dealership where he has worked for fifty years. The only difference is that he takes more vacations. Alex is eighty-four years young.

8

NOURISHING THE EMOTIONAL

Renew

Stop for a minute and look at your present circumstances. Are you satisfied with your life and how you are feeling? Are you growing, learning and taking care of yourself? Or do you feel you don't have anything exciting to look forward to?

If that's the case, you're stuck. The good news is that this is an excellent place to start, because you can't improve your life unless you clearly understand that something has to change.

Is it your physical well-being? Your state of mind? Your lack of spirituality? Do you even know where to begin to make changes? Take longer than a minute, take as long as you need to think about what you can do to get out of the glue that's keeping you stuck.

Being stuck brings a feeling of hopelessness. Luckily, there are ways to get unstuck and be free to live your dreams. It's like being inside a dark room or a closet and all you need is for someone to open the door and let in a little light.

I remember that feeling. I was fifty-nine during the hard economic times in Argentina with inflation out of control and my businesses in jeopardy. There was no way I could stop the destruction of my lifestyle and the devaluation of my properties.

I was a household name throughout Latin America. I had beauty spas and beauty schools all over Argentina and a successful product line. More than 15,000 estheticians graduated from my first School of Feminine Esthetics. Our headquarters were in Buenos Aires with franchises in major cities.

Hundreds of articles had been written about me and by me. I wrote three books that were used as text books in beauty schools. One of them, *The Encyclopedia of Esthetics*, was in four volumes.

Then, like many people in Argentina, I suffered the effects of rampant inflation and an unstable marketplace. And my beloved Alberto died. I lost my husband, my best friend and my business partner.

It felt as if I had no future. I was completely stuck in a dark room. That's when I decided to move to the United States, leave everything behind and start afresh.

I wanted to celebrate my sixtieth birthday with a new beginning in a country where economic ups and downs were not so strongly felt. Coming to a place where no one knew me and starting a new career from scratch at sixty wasn't easy, but at least I got unstuck and I had some relatives here.

I had to be creative and the light that came into my room was the help I received from my family. My brother and my sister were already in America. Susana said I could live with her rent-free for six months and my brother and sister-in-law connected me with all their Argentinean friends who became my first clients in Los Angeles. They also helped me get Rodrigo here by sponsoring his visa application.

Second chances can be the best remedy for the worst of times. I forgot about my celebrity status and left the headaches of running a large company behind me. I opened a small spa in Los Angeles and adjusted my product line to meet FDA standards. So began my new life.

Sometimes it takes what seems like a catastrophe to shake your world and provide the impetus to start over. Mine gave me the chance to rejuvenate and create a much happier way of life. I am so grateful that what felt like tragedy at the time happened to me.

Hopefully, if you feel stuck, it won't take so much drama for you to get out of the glue that's holding you back. Perhaps a dear friend talks to you and gives good advice, or you learn a new skill, adopt a pet or even reading this book will inspire you to get unstuck.

Update and uplift

Revolution is about change. But change doesn't need to be revolutionary. It can happen by making small shifts.

Transformation is the way life works. You can't avoid it, so you may as well enjoy the ride.

Change never stops, for good or bad. When you think, *I am too old to change*, you're saying, *I am too old to change into something better.*

If you don't take action, change will happen without your consent, by itself and in the direction of hopelessness. And the terrible truth is that when you get to that point, you're not living, you're just lasting.

So here you are, at the beginning of the rest of your life (this can happen at any age) and you have to make a decision: living or lasting? Are you joining the "Stay Young Revolution" or "The Giving Up On Yourself Brigade?"

When you exercise regularly your muscles change, your posture changes and you breathe better. These are all positive changes. For me, in my ninetieth year, my favorite ways to exercise are water aerobics and walking on the treadmill. Find something you enjoy and get moving.

When you join a travel group, your mind expands and your outlook on the world changes. You are living, not lasting. These are all positive changes.

Starting a new activity or learning to do the thing you always wanted but never got around to will make a positive change in your brain and you will feel rejuvenated.

Revise your attitude about change and make sure positive changes come into play. Above all, keep telling yourself: *I can make myself happy. I don't mind a few changes in the right direction.*

Be the controller of your own destiny.

The world's greatest endurance swimmer is Diana Nyad. In 2013, on her fifth attempt and at age sixty-four, she became the first person to swim from Cuba to Florida without the protection of a shark cage.

Bernice Gordon is the world's oldest professional crossword puzzle constructor. She sold her first puzzle to the *New York Times* in 1952 and still compiles a new puzzle every day. She's ninety-nine!

I believe that anything we focus on has a tendency to grow. Focus on negativity and you get more of it. Focus on fear and you get more fearful. Focus on loving yourself and others, and the feeling of love will extend to everything that surrounds you.

It seems that intention is the energy that binds our heart and our mind. What you project emotionally is what the universe projects back. The best way to stay young is to clean up your feelings by eliminating all the ones that set you back.

Right now, as you analyze what is on your plate

emotionally, try to distinguish negative energies like jealousy, envy, depression and self-pity. Look as objectively as possible to realize what is separating you from happiness and bravely confront those feelings so you understand what's causing them.

What will it take to change the darkness into light? There are many ways, ranging from a bite of chocolate to a series of sessions with your psychotherapist.

Do not let the darkness linger. Transform it into your bliss.

As I write this chapter, there is some controversy at the 2014 Sochi Winter Olympics. A former hurdler, Lolo Jones, is well known as a track and field athlete. She never won a gold medal, but she came pretty close. Then she became a member of a United States bobsled team. She switched because track and field is a lonely pursuit and didn't make her happy. She wanted to be part of a team, to share the feelings of participating in a common effort and to support, and be supported by, her teammates.

Whatever other reasons motivated her to take up a team sport, the lesson I see here is that she had the courage to confront the cause of her unhappiness and do something about it.

9

NOURISHING THE SPIRITUAL

Religion

This important leg to the table of our lives can look very different for each one of us. To me, religion is a matter of study, not of faith. My ancestors were free thinkers and Judaism was just a tradition for them, not a religious practice. My parents strongly believed in freedom of choice in all matters and showed it in every aspect of their lives.

The parents of one of my relatives, having the same type of freedom of choice in mind, decided not to have their baby boy circumcised, feeling it was such an important decision that he should make it himself when he was an adult. Later in life, he did exercise that freedom of choice when he became a prominent member of a temple in California. Good for him.

I call my spiritual beliefs the energy soup. It is like a minestrone soup where the chicken broth is the general energy that represents our environment and the different pieces that float around – of various textures, flavors and colors – represent all the parts that comprise our universe, each with its own form of energy. Each energy plays a role in our lives – high energy, low energy, good energy and not-so-good energy – they all interact to keep us going.

I also like to live in the present, combining the energies that circulate around me from my work, friends, thoughts and the many circumstances beyond my control. The soup tastes different every day. I find that a fascinating and easy way to understand how energy flows. Create your own soup.

Meditation

A great way to connect with the spiritual side of your being is to meditate. It's something I highly recommend for every SYR.

Personally, I meditate every day, practicing a self-designed variety. I find a quiet spot, sit down on the floor or a chair, cut off any thoughts of daily concerns, breathe deeply and rhythmically and get ready to take the plunge. This is a different form of relaxation than just taking a nap, although both napping and meditating are forms of renewing the spiritual and emotional energies.

In meditation, I have the feeling of jumping into a luminous place similar to a big pool of water in the sunlight. I imagine myself as a dolphin, swimming up and down, playing in the water. It's a deep, peaceful and joyous experience that erases any worries and preoccupations. For about fifteen to twenty minutes every day, my soul is ageless and I come back to reality fully recharged.

There are dozens of specific styles of meditation or meditative practices. You probably already know about some of them or maybe you feel inspired to do some research. A wise woman told me that anyone who says they are too busy to meditate once a day should do it twice a day.

So, my fellow SYRs, take a look at your spiritual world and make sure it's uplifting or at least that you have a pretty good one, so the four legs of your life table are reassuringly even.

MARTHA WEINSTEIN

10

DRIVING MISS MARTHA

Acceptance

For some senior citizens, it can feel depressing and a bitter blow that they can no longer drive or travel. If you want an excuse to be depressed, there are many good ones out there. You have to always look on the positive side and accept some changes as time goes by.

The Serenity Prayer is so relevant here and inspirational to us all, even if we're not involved in a 12-Step Program:

Grant me the serenity
To accept the things I cannot change,
Courage to change the things I can,
And the wisdom to know the difference.

One of the biggest fears of aging is no longer being able to drive. There are stories of people of a certain age making mistakes and confusing the pedals, pushing for the gas when they should have pressed the brake.

That happened to me. I was driving to a new hairdresser and he came outside the salon signaling me to park somewhere, and I got flustered. I pressed the gas pedal instead of the brake and hit a wall. But that happened when my age definitely wasn't a factor. I was seventy-two and driving perfectly well up until that point where I became momentarily confused, which can happen to anyone at any age.

Nothing more serious than a few scratches on the car and the wall happened in my little accident, but there are cases where people and property are seriously damaged. But don't wait for a terrible accident to stop driving. When you feel the time has come, your internal voice or conscience will tell you. Listen to it. We should all be responsible enough to know when we no longer feel safe. I think every case is different, though. Some brains function better at ninety than others at sixty, so I don't believe there should be an age limit for driving.

Living car-free doesn't have to be a negative thing. You can save a lot of money when you add up the costs of leasing or purchase payments, insurance, registration, repairs, gas and parking. Do the math and you'll be surprised.

My son, Rodrigo, is in the real estate business. He explained to me how much money I'd save by not driving and using his preferred choice instead.

Uber is available in many countries and cities. It's an app that summons a car to take you anywhere you want. You can't book in advance, but can order one within a few minutes via your phone. You sign up for the service in advance and the fare is automatically taken out of your bank account or charged to your credit card. You can use it as often or as seldom as you like and there is no tipping.

The cars are impeccable and the drivers courteous. They open the door for you and make sure you are comfortable. I've found them to be cheaper than taxis.

If you can have such an excellent service without the expense and other aggravations of having a car, you can reach the conclusion that it's pretty easy to live car-free and away from the dangers of driving. Other car services are available, of course, so find the one that best suits your needs.

To stay as young as possible at any age, you always have to listen to your internal voice. One day you might find it's no longer a pleasure to make international flights.

Going through the aggravation at the airport and sharing confined spaces with a lot of other people is stressful to me now, so I no longer like to fly for holidays. I want to be driven somewhere not too far away by someone else, without the stress of flying.

I would fly for business and to visit family, but not for pleasure. I have many happy memories from vacations to recall instead.

There may also come a time when you don't want to cook any more. That happened to me early in life. I'm not fond of cooking. In my younger days, I could feed my family but I wouldn't say it was cooking. When I have to feed myself, I can't call it cooking either. I am fond of eating out and always have been.

Look for solutions to problems that can make you feel good about yourself. That's one of the most important parts about staying young and feeling good. Don't dwell on the negative aspects of anything.

Make sure the relationship with yourself and others is based on acceptance. It might take a little compassion, a little forgiveness, and a lot of flexibility, but if there is no acceptance there will be no peace.

When I was a little girl, about three years old, my mother wanted me to be brave and sleep alone in the dark in my bedroom far down the corridor. I didn't feel so brave, but luckily I had a loving nanny who was compassionate with me. Every night when she put me to bed, I begged her, "Ya-Ya, please don't forget to keep the light on in the corridor." Now I live by myself, but I never forget to leave the light on in the corridor. I sleep so well with that little light burning outside my bedroom.

Light has always been important in my life. Light to receive, light to give, light from anywhere to see better, feel better and to open our hearts and minds to clear the past and dissolve darkness, to create some clarity out of confusion. And many times to make a connection with another human being, our own angels and demons, plus, of course, with that bigger light that controls the universe.

Connection is so important. Rituals can sometimes create

connection.

There was a priest in the Middle Ages who arrived at a poor community in Italy at the end of the month, the twenty-ninth. The villagers wanted to make him feel welcome and provide a good meal, but all they had left were potatoes.

They wondered what on earth they could do to make the potatoes into something more sophisticated and interesting. They came up with a combination of potato and flour to make little dumplings with a tasty sauce to accompany it.

The priest was grateful and said, "I will bless these dumplings and call them gnocchi. Make sure you eat them on the twenty-ninth of every month and you will always have enough money the next month to pay all your bills."

Because there are so many Italian immigrants in Argentina who continued the tradition, eating gnocchi on the twenty-ninth of each month almost became a national sport. I brought the tradition with me to the United States and whenever I meet with my Argentinean and American friends on the twenty-ninth, we carry out the same ritual and put money under our plates. There's the little secret to the success of the ceremony, not only eating the gnocchi but taking a bank note, folding it in a special way to make a knot, and placing it under your plate. When you've finished eating, while it's still warm, you put it back in your purse or wallet and that guarantees you will pay your bills next month. You can never spend that note because if you spend it, it loses its magic.

I think simple rituals are a good thing, a good excuse for friends to come together and have something in common that bonds them. I've been doing it for the thirty years I've lived in America and I always have had enough money to pay my bills every month. That's most likely because I work hard, but I don't want to take the risk and miss my gnocchi ritual, nor the connection with my friends.

To my great advantage, I have always had friends much younger than myself. My best friend Patito (it means little duck) is forty-five years younger than me and we have been friends for thirty years.

I was sixty and Patito was fourteen when we first met, but somehow we clicked from day one. She is the person I call when I am conflicted because she has this magical power to ease my stress when I talk to her. After thirty years, Patito knows me well. I highly recommend to all SYRs that you keep making new friendships, to get excited, rejuvenated and interested in all kinds of lives.

To stay young, you have to recognize all the different ways available to let energy flow through the channels designed for that purpose. A clear image comes to mind when we talk about meridians.

In Chinese medicine, meridians are a group of lines in the body around which energy circulates. Illness occurs when the regular flow along those lines is interrupted and the energy gets blocked. To restore the normal flow, Chinese medicine uses acupuncture, sometimes acupressure, both forms of intervention to offset the blockage.

There are other forms of so-called energy healing known as alternative medicine worth exploring to find what works for you.

A more elaborate school of energy healing called "The Reconnection" opens new insights into the concept of meridians. This Western approach, based on ancient Chinese practices, supports the notion of meridians extending outside our bodies and reaching far into the universe. It's said that a much more intense healing can occur if we reconnect with those extended meridians and let the process develop.

The promoter and developer of this idea is a chiropractor, Dr. Eric Pearl. You can Google him if his ideas intrigue you. I like the idea of reconnecting to energy sources of any kind. I believe there are many different ones that are reachable: physical energy, emotional energy, mental energy and spiritual energy. All of them are contributing to who we are and can help us become who we want to be.

So, my dear friends and fellow Stay Young Revolutionaries, keep moving, keep smiling, eat healthily, cleanse, exfoliate, moisturize, connect and have lots of fun. Make sure your life story is a long, happy, healthy and beautiful one, taking your inner child out to play as often as possible.

Let's spread the revolution.

When I arrived in the United States aged sixty, my son Rodrigo (who has always supported my endeavors) said, "Mother, how much longer are you going to work?"

I said, "Five years."

Five years later, he would ask me again and I would reply, "Five years."

Every five years it felt like I was renewing the lease on the possibility of my still being productive.

This year, when I celebrate my ninetieth birthday, I am sure Rodrigo will ask me the same question again. This time, I have a dilemma. Do I dare say five more years again? Who knows?

Long live the revolution!

ABOUT THE CO-AUTHOR

Claire Fordham is a British journalist and TV producer. Her acclaimed book, *Plus One: A Year In The Life of a Hollywood Nobody* inspired the film *The Making Of Plus One* starring Jennifer Tilly, Amanda Plummer and Geraldine Chaplin. Claire is a proud member of The Stay Young Revolution. She lives in Los Angeles.

MARTHA WEINSTEIN

The fear of aging is one of the most pervasive sources of stress in our culture. Martha Weinstein's Stay Young Revolution is the cure for the aging blues. Early in life, Martha developed her own brand of age arresters, intuitively combining good nutrition, exercise, skincare and integrated medicine with her great sense of humor. This book should be in the same category as *Chicken Soup for the Soul* and widely translated for people all over the world.

L. E – Executive

Like an elixir of wisdom, Martha's encouraging words made me rejuvenate. My advice, drink the elixir.

A.B - Homeopath

I understand myself better and like myself more since I joined the Stay Young Revolution. Thanks, Martha.

R.I.V. - Entrepreneur

I will be 91 this year and I am still following Martha's regimen for beautiful longevity every day. No wonder people tell me "you never change."

M.F.- Author

There are many books on longevity but none has the freshness of personal experience. The anecdotes from Martha's own life and the stories of people she knows are splendid examples of what it means to stay young.

P.R.- Energy Healer

MARTHA WEINSTEIN